I0210131

47 Home Remedy Juice Recipes for Ovarian Cancer:

Vitamin Packed Recipes That Will Give Your Body What It Needs to Fight Cancer Cells

By

Joe Correa CSN

COPYRIGHT

© 2017 Live Stronger Faster Inc.

All rights reserved

Reproduction or translation of any part of this work beyond that permitted by section 107 or 108 of the 1976 United States Copyright Act without the permission of the copyright owner is unlawful.

This publication is designed to provide accurate and authoritative information in regard to the subject matter covered. It is sold with the understanding that neither the author nor the publisher is engaged in rendering medical advice. If medical advice or assistance is needed, consult with a doctor. This book is considered a guide and should not be used in any way detrimental to your health. Consult with a physician before starting this nutritional plan to make sure it's right for you.

ACKNOWLEDGEMENTS

This book is dedicated to my friends and family that have had mild or serious illnesses so that you may find a solution and make the necessary changes in your life.

47 Home Remedy Juice Recipes for Ovarian Cancer:

Vitamin Packed Recipes That Will Give Your Body What It Needs to Fight Cancer Cells

By

Joe Correa CSN

CONTENTS

Copyright

Acknowledgements

About The Author

Introduction

47 Home Remedy Juice Recipes for Ovarian Cancer: Vitamin Packed Recipes That Will Give Your Body What It Needs to Fight Cancer Cells

Additional Titles from This Author

ABOUT THE AUTHOR

After years of Research, I honestly believe in the positive effects that proper nutrition can have over the body and mind. My knowledge and experience has helped me live healthier throughout the years and which I have shared with family and friends. The more you know about eating and drinking healthier, the sooner you will want to change your life and eating habits.

Nutrition is a key part in the process of being healthy and living longer so get started today. The first step is the most important and the most significant.

INTRODUCTION

47 Home Remedy Juice Recipes for Ovarian Cancer: Vitamin Packed Recipes That Will Give Your Body What It Needs to Fight Cancer Cells

By Joe Correa CSN

When we talk about ovarian cancer preventing foods, we simply have to mention juices. This is the easiest way to give your body all the nutrients it needs to stay healthy. Besides, they are easy to make and can fit into anybody's budget and schedule. This is why I have created this healthy collection of delicious juice recipes that will help you fight off ovarian cancer.

Juicing is not something new. It is an old yet very popular way of consuming multiple fruits and vegetables at the same time. This powerful method has been proven to improve your immune system and overall health within a couple of minutes of preparation. When using the right ingredients, the results are simply amazing!

Ovarian cancer is a serious disease and it is the fifth leading cause of cancer-related death among women. These horrible statistics simply can't be ignored and the best way to prevent this is to start taking care of your health through food. Juice recipes that are based on good and healthy ingredients will strengthen your immune system, restore intestinal integrity, and provide essential nutrients ranging from amino acids to vitamins and minerals.

Today, the popularity of juicing fruits and vegetables is greater than ever before. This positive trend has reminded us of all the health benefits raw foods have. We may or may not have the time to eat healthy, but the fact is that everybody has a couple of minutes to prepare a delicious juice in the morning and start the day in the best possible manner. Returning to these old fashioned healing methods will bring us many benefits.

When we talk about ovarian cancer, the best possible ingredients are avocado, cabbage, bell peppers, tomatoes, asparagus, green tea, grapefruits, ginger, and berries. These powerful ingredients should be the basis of your ovarian cancer-fighting juices.

Juicing is not some new diet trend but a powerful healing tool you can easily implement in your daily routine. It's one of the best things you can do for yourself and your entire family! Stop ovarian cancer now by using these unique recipes.

47 HOME REMEDY JUICE RECIPES FOR OVARIAN CANCER: VITAMIN PACKED RECIPES THAT WILL GIVE YOUR BODY WHAT IT NEEDS TO FIGHT CANCER CELLS

1. Lettuce Avocado Juice

Ingredients:

2 cups of Romaine lettuce, torn

1 cup of avocado, cubed

1 cup of fresh kale, torn

1 whole kiwi, peeled

1 whole cucumber, sliced

Preparation:

Combine lettuce and kale in a large colander. Wash thoroughly under cold running water and torn into small pieces. Set aside.

Peel the avocado and cut lengthwise in half. Remove the pit and cut into small cubes. Fill the measuring cup and reserve the rest for later.

Peel the kiwi and cut lengthwise in half. Set aside.

Wash the cucumber and cut into thin slices. Fill the measuring cup and reserve the rest for later.

Now, combine lettuce, kale, avocado, kiwi, and cucumber in a juicer and process until juiced. Transfer to a serving glass and add some ice before serving.

Enjoy!

Nutritional information per serving: Kcal: 304, Protein: 9.8g, Carbs: 42.8g, Fats: 23.6g

2.   Broccoli Cabbage Juice

Ingredients:

2 cups of broccoli, chopped

1 cup of green cabbage, torn

1 small green apple, cored

1 cup of cauliflower, chopped

2 tbsp of spring onions, chopped

¼ tsp of turmeric, ground

1 oz of water

Preparation:

Wash the broccoli and trim off the outer layers. Chop into small pieces and fill the measuring cup. Reserve the rest for later.

Wash the cabbage thoroughly under cold running water and drain. Torn into small pieces and set aside.

Wash the apple and cut lengthwise in half. Remove the core and cut into bite-sized pieces. Set aside.

Wash the cauliflower and trim off the outer leaves. Chop into small pieces and fill the measuring cup. Reserve the rest in the refrigerator.

Rinse the onion stalk and chop into small pieces. Set aside.

Now, combine broccoli, cabbage, apple, cauliflower, and onions in a juicer and process until juiced.

Transfer to a serving glass and stir in the turmeric and water. Refrigerate for 10 minutes before serving.

Nutritional information per serving: Kcal: 127, Protein: 6.6g, Carbs: 37.9g, Fats: 1.1g

3.   Green Tea Juice

Ingredients:

1 tsp of green tea powder

2 cups of spinach, torn

1 cup of watercress, torn

1 cup of kale, torn

1 cup of Swiss chard, torn

¼ tsp of ginger, ground

1 oz of water

Preparation:

Combine, spinach, watercress, kale, and Swiss chard in a large colander. Wash thoroughly under cold running water. Slightly drain and torn into small pieces.

Place the tea powder in a small bowl. Add 3 tbsp of hot water and stir well. Set aside for 3 minutes.

Now, combine spinach, watercress, kale, and Swiss chard in a juicer and process until juiced. Transfer to a serving glass and stir in the ginger and water.

Refrigerate for 20 minutes before serving.

Enjoy!

Nutritional information per serving: Kcal: 87, Protein: 16.3g, Carbs: 22.9g, Fats: 2.4g

4.   Asparagus Bell Pepper Juice

Ingredients:

1 cup of asparagus, trimmed

1 large green bell pepper, chopped

1 cup of celery, chopped

¼ tsp of turmeric, ground

¼ tsp of ginger, ground

1 oz of water

Preparation:

Wash the asparagus and trim off the woody ends. Cut into small pieces and fill the measuring cup. Reserve the rest in the refrigerator.

Wash the bell pepper and cut lengthwise in half. Remove the stem and seeds. Chop into small pieces and set aside.

Wash the celery and chop into small pieces. Set aside.

Now, combine asparagus, pepper, and celery in a juicer and process until well juiced. Transfer to a serving glass and stir in the turmeric, ginger, and water.

Add some ice and serve immediately.

Enjoy!

Nutritional information per serving: Kcal: 48, Protein: 5.1g, Carbs: 15.8g, Fats: 0.6g

5.   Grapefruit Orange Juice

Ingredients:

1 whole grapefruit, peeled

1 large orange, peeled

1 cup of cucumber, sliced

1 cup of papaya, chopped

¼ tsp of cinnamon, ground

2 tbsp of coconut water

Preparation:

Peel the grapefruit and orange. Divide into wedges. Cut each wedge in half and set aside.

Wash the cucumber and cut into thin slices. Fill the measuring cup and reserve the rest for later.

Peel the papaya and cut into small chunks. Fill the measuring cup and reserve the rest in the refrigerator.

Now, combine grapefruit, orange, cucumber, and papaya in a juicer and process until well juiced.

Transfer to a serving glass and stir in the cinnamon and coconut water.

Refrigerate for 10 minutes before serving.

Nutritional information per serving: Kcal: 214, Protein: 4.6g, Carbs: 65.4g, Fats: 1g

6.   Cauliflower Carrot Juice

Ingredients:

1 cup of cauliflower, chopped

2 large carrots, sliced

1 large radish, chopped

1 cup of turnip greens, torn

¼ tsp of ginger, ground

2 oz of water

Preparation:

Trim off the outer leaves of the cauliflower. Wash it and chop into small pieces. Fill the measuring cup and reserve the rest for later.

Wash and peel the carrots. Cut into thin slices and set aside.

Wash the radish and chop into small pieces. Set aside.

Wash the turnip greens thoroughly under cold running water. Drain and torn into small pieces. Set aside.

Now, combine cauliflower, carrots, radish, and turnip greens in a juicer and process until juiced. Transfer to a serving glass and stir in the ginger and water.

Add some ice and serve immediately.

Nutritional information per serving: Kcal: 75, Protein: 4.3g, Carbs: 23.3g, Fats: 0.8g

7.   Pomegranate Banana Juice

Ingredients:

1 cup of pomegranate seeds

1 large banana, chopped

1 small Granny Smith's apple, cored

1 cup of raspberries

¼ tsp of ginger, ground

Preparation:

Cut the top of the pomegranate fruit using a sharp paring knife. Slice down to each of the white membranes inside of the fruit. Pop the seeds into a measuring cup and set aside.

Peel the banana and cut into small pieces. Set aside.

Wash the apple and cut lengthwise in half. Remove the core and cut into bite-sized pieces. Set aside.

Rinse the raspberries under cold running water using a colander. Drain and set aside.

Now, combine pomegranate seeds, banana, apple, and raspberries in a juicer and process until juiced. Transfer to a serving glass and stir in the ginger.

Add some ice and serve immediately.

Nutritional information per serving: Kcal: 265, Protein: 5.1g, Carbs: 81.6g, Fats: 2.5g

8.   Artichoke Spinach Juice

Ingredients:

1 large artichoke, chopped

1 cup of fresh spinach, torn

1 cup of green cabbage, torn

1 cup of avocado, cubed

¼ tsp of turmeric, ground

Preparation:

Trim off the outer layers of the artichoke using a sharp paring knife. Cut into bite-sized pieces and set aside.

Combine spinach and cabbage in a large colander. Wash thoroughly under cold running water. Drain and torn into small pieces. Set aside.

Peel the avocado and cut lengthwise in half. Remove the pit and cut into small cubes. Fill the measuring cup and reserve the rest in the refrigerator.

Now, combine artichoke, spinach, cabbage, and avocado in a juicer and process until juiced. Transfer to a serving glass and stir in the turmeric.

Refrigerate for 10 minutes before serving.

Nutritional information per serving: Kcal: 282, Protein: 15.4g, Carbs: 42.6g, Fats: 23.2g

9.   Pineapple Blackberry Juice

Ingredients:

1 cup of pineapple, chunked

1 cup of blackberries

1 cup of fresh mint, chopped

1 whole lime, peeled

2 oz of coconut water

Preparation:

Using a sharp paring knife, cut the top of the pineapple. Gently remove all hard skin and slice it into thin slices. Fill the measuring cup and reserve the rest for later.

Place the blackberries in a large colander. Rinse thoroughly under cold running water. Drain and set aside.

Wash the mint and drain. Chop into small pieces and set aside.

Peel the lime and cut lengthwise in half. Set aside.

Now, combine pineapple, blackberries, mint, and lime in a juicer. Process until well juiced and transfer to a serving glass.

Stir in the coconut water and add few ice cubes before serving. Enjoy!

Nutritional information per serving: Kcal: 125, Protein: 4g, Carbs: 42.9g, Fats: 1.2g

10.   Pumpkin Chard Juice

Ingredients:

1 cup of pumpkin, chopped

1 cup of Swiss chard, torn

1 medium-sized zucchini, chopped

1 cup of cucumber, sliced

¼ tsp of ginger, ground

1 oz of water

Preparation:

Cut the top of a pumpkin. Cut lengthwise in half and then scrape out the seeds. Cut one large wedge and peel it. Cut into small cubes and fill the measuring cup. Reserve the rest in the refrigerator.

Wash the Swiss chard thoroughly under cold running water. Drain and torn into small pieces. Set aside.

Wash the zucchini and cut into thin slices. Set aside.

Wash the cucumber and cut into slices. Fill the measuring cup and reserve the rest for later.

Now, combine pumpkin, Swiss chard, zucchini, and cucumber in a juicer and process until juiced. Transfer to a serving glass and stir in the ginger and water.

Serve cold.

Nutritional information per serving: Kcal: 65, Protein: 4.5g, Carbs: 16.8g, Fats: 0.8g

11.   Lemon Mango Juice

Ingredients:

2 whole lemons, peeled and halved

1 cup of mango, chunked

1 whole grapefruit, peeled and wedged

1 small Granny Smith's apple, cored

¼ tsp of ginger, ground

Preparation:

Peel the lemons and cut each lengthwise in half. Set aside.

Peel the mango and cut into chunks. Fill the measuring cup and reserve the rest for later. Set aside.

Peel the grapefruit and divide into wedges. Cut each wedge in half and set aside.

Wash the apple and cut lengthwise in half. Remove the core and cut into bite-sized pieces. Set aside.

Now, combine lemon, mango, grapefruit, and apple in a juicer and process until juiced. Transfer to a serving glass and stir in the ginger.

Add few ice cubes and serve immediately.

Enjoy!

Nutritional information per serving: Kcal: 65, Protein: 4.5g, Carbs: 16.8g, Fats: 0.8g

12.   Beet-Orange Juice

Ingredients:

1 cup of beets, trimmed and sliced

1 large orange, peeled

1 cup of black grapes

1 whole apricot, pitted

1 tbsp of coconut water

Preparation:

Wash the beets and trim off the green parts. Cut into thin slices and fill the measuring cup. Reserve the rest for later.

Peel the orange and divide into wedges. Cut each wedge in half and set aside.

Rinse the grapes and remove the stems. Set aside.

Wash the apricot and cut lengthwise in half. Remove the pit and cut into small pieces. Set aside.

Now, combine beets, orange, grapes, and apricots in a juicer and process until well juiced. Transfer to a serving glass and stir in the coconut water.

Add some ice and serve immediately.

Nutritional information per serving: Kcal: 184, Protein: 4.9g, Carbs: 54.3g, Fats: 0.9g

13. Cherry Plum Juice

Ingredients:

1 cup of cherries, pitted

2 whole plums, pitted and chopped

1 small green apple, cored

1 cup of strawberries, chopped

1 tbsp of coconut water

¼ tsp of ginger, ground

Preparation:

Wash the cherries thoroughly using a large colander. Drain and cut each in half. Remove the pits and cut into small pieces. Set aside.

Wash the plums and cut in half. Remove the pits and cut into small bite-sized pieces. Set aside.

Wash the apple and cut lengthwise in half. Remove the core and cut into small pieces. Set aside.

Wash the strawberries and remove the stems. Cut into small pieces and fill the measuring cup. Reserve the rest for later. Set aside.

Now, combine cherries, plums, apple, and strawberries in a juicer and process until juiced. Transfer to a serving glass and stir in the coconut water and ginger.

Add some crushed ice and serve immediately.

Nutritional information per serving: Kcal: 236, Protein: 4.2g, Carbs: 70.3g, Fats: 1.3g

14.   Pear Cranberry Juice

Ingredients:

1 large pear, chopped

1 cup of cranberries

1 whole lemon, peeled

1 cup of watermelon, chunked

¼ tsp of cinnamon, ground

1 oz of water

Preparation:

Wash the pear and cut in half. Remove the core and cut into small pieces. Set aside.

Place the cranberries in a colander and rinse under cold running water. Drain and set aside.

Peel the lemon and cut lengthwise in half. Set aside.

Cut the watermelon in half. Cut one large wedge and wrap the rest in a plastic foil and refrigerate. Peel the slice and cut into small cubes. Remove the pits and fill the measuring cup. Set aside.

Now, combine pear, cranberries, lemon, and watermelon in a juicer and process until well juiced. Transfer to a serving glass and stir in the cinnamon and water.

Refrigerate for 10 minutes before serving.

Nutritional information per serving: Kcal: 186, Protein: 2.8g, Carbs: 64.1g, Fats: 0.8g

15.   Strawberry Avocado Juice

Ingredients:

1 cup of strawberries, chopped

1 cup of avocado, cubed

1 large peach, chopped

1 large Granny Smith's apple, cored

¼ tsp of cinnamon, ground

¼ tsp of ginger, ground

2 tsp of coconut water

Preparation:

Wash the strawberries and remove the stems. Cut into bite-sized pieces and fill the measuring cup. Reserve the rest for later.

Peel the avocado and cut in half. Remove the pit and cut into small cubes. Fill the measuring cup and reserve the rest for later.

Wash the peach and cut lengthwise in half. Remove the pit and cut into bite-sized pieces. Set aside.

Wash the apple and cut in half. Remove the core and chop into small pieces. Set aside.

Now, combine strawberries, avocado, peach, and apple in a juicer and process until juiced. Transfer to a serving glass and stir in the cinnamon, ginger, and coconut water.

Refrigerate for 15 minutes before serving.

Nutritional information per serving: Kcal: 386, Protein: 6.5g, Carbs: 68.6g, Fats: 23.2g

16.   Celery Basil Juice

Ingredients:

1 cup of celery, chopped

1 cup of fresh basil, torn

1 cup of cucumber, sliced

1 whole lime, peeled

1 medium-sized apple, cored

Preparation:

Wash the celery and cut into small pieces. Set aside.

Wash the basil thoroughly under cold running water. Drain and torn into small pieces. Set aside.

Wash the cucumber and cut into thin slices. Fill the measuring cup and reserve the rest for later. Set aside.

Peel the lime and cut lengthwise in half. Set aside.

Wash the apple and cut lengthwise in half. Remove the core and cut into bite-sized pieces. Set aside.

Now, combine celery, basil, cucumber, lime, and apple in a juicer and process until well juiced. Transfer to a serving glass and add some crushed ice.

Serve immediately.

Nutritional information per serving: Kcal: 109, Protein: 2.7g, Carbs: 31.9g, Fats: 0.7g

17. Orange Plum Juice

Ingredients:

1 large orange, peeled

1 whole plum, chopped

1 cup of cantaloupe, chopped

1 cup of fresh mint, torn

¼ tsp of turmeric, ground

¼ tsp of ginger, ground

Preparation:

Peel the orange and divide into wedges. Cut each wedge in half and set aside.

Wash the plum and cut in half. Remove the pit and chop into small pieces. Set aside.

Cut the cantaloupe in half. Scoop out the seeds and flesh. Cut and peel one large wedge. Chop into chunks and fill the measuring cup. Reserve the rest of the cantaloupe in a refrigerator.

Wash the mint thoroughly under cold running water. Torn into small pieces and set aside.

Now, combine orange, plum, cantaloupe, and mint in a juicer and process until juiced. Transfer to a serving glass and stir in the turmeric and ginger.

Add some ice and serve immediately.

Enjoy!

Nutritional information per serving: Kcal: 151, Protein: 4.4g, Carbs: 45.6g, Fats: 0.9g

18.   Fennel Collard Greens Juice

Ingredients:

1 whole fennel bulb, chopped

1 cup of collard greens, chopped

1 cup of cucumber, sliced

1 whole lemon, peeled

1 oz of water

¼ tsp of cayenne pepper, ground

Preparation:

Trim off the fennel bulb and remove the green parts. Wash the bulb and cut into small pieces. Set aside.

Rinse the collard greens under cold running water. Drain and chop into small pieces. Set aside.

Wash the cucumber and cut into thin slices. Fill the measuring cup and reserve the rest for later. Set aside.

Peel the lemon and cut lengthwise in half. Set aside.

Now, combine fennel, collard greens, cucumber, and lemon in a juicer and process until juiced. Transfer to a serving glass and stir in the water and cayenne pepper.

Refrigerate for 20 minutes before serving.

Enjoy!

Nutritional information per serving: Kcal: 68, Protein: 4.9g, Carbs: 26.3g, Fats: 0.9g

19.   Mango Peach Juice

Ingredients:

1 cup of mango, chunked

1 medium-sized peach, chopped

1 large banana, chunked

1 large orange, peeled

¼ tsp of cinnamon, ground

Preparation:

Peel the mango and cut into small chunks. Fill the measuring cup and reserve the rest for later. Set aside.

Wash the peach and cut lengthwise in half. Remove the pit and cut into small pieces. Set aside.

Peel the banana and cut into small chunks. Set aside.

Peel the orange and divide into wedges. Cut each wedge in half and set aside.

Now, combine mango, peach, banana, and orange in a juicer. Process until well juiced. Transfer to a serving glass and stir in the cinnamon.

Add some crushed ice and serve immediately.

Enjoy!

Nutritional information per serving: Kcal: 313, Protein: 5.9g, Carbs: 91.7g, Fats: 1.6g

20.   Tomato Spinach Juice

Ingredients:

1 medium-sized tomato, chopped

1 cup of fresh spinach, torn

1 whole lemon, peeled

1 large red bell pepper, chopped

1 tsp of rosemary, finely chopped

Preparation:

Wash the tomato and place in a small bowl. Chop into small pieces and reserve the tomato juice while cutting. Set aside.

Wash the spinach thoroughly under cold running water. Drain and torn into small pieces. Set aside.

Peel the lemon and cut lengthwise in half. Set aside.

Wash the bell pepper and cut in half. Remove the stem and seeds. Cut into small pieces and set aside.

Now, combine tomato, spinach, lemon, and bell pepper in a juicer and process until juiced. Transfer to a serving glass and stir in the rosemary.

Add few ice cubes and serve immediately.

Nutritional information per serving: Kcal: 92, Protein: 9.3g, Carbs: 27.7g, Fats: 1.7g

21.   Avocado Lettuce Juice

Ingredients:

1 cup of avocado, chunked

1 cup of red leaf lettuce, shredded

1 large banana, sliced

½ cup of strawberries, chopped

1 small Red Delicious apple, cored

¼ tsp of cinnamon, ground

Preparation:

Peel the avocado and cut lengthwise in half. Remove the pit and chop into small pieces. Set aside.

Wash the lettuce thoroughly under cold running water. Drain and chop into small pieces. Set aside.

Peel the banana and chop into small pieces. Set aside.

Wash the strawberries and remove the stems. Cut into bite-sized pieces and fill the measuring cup. Set aside.

Now, combine avocado, lettuce, banana, and strawberries in a juicer and process until juiced. Transfer to a serving glass and stir in the cinnamon.

Add some ice and serve immediately.

Enjoy!

Nutritional information per serving: Kcal: 405, Protein: 5.7g, Carbs: 72.2g, Fats: 23.1g

22. Apricot Strawberry Juice

Ingredients:

1 cup of apricots, chopped

1 cup of strawberries, chopped

1 cup of celery, chopped

1 small Golden Delicious apple, cored

¼ tsp of cinnamon, ground

Preparation:

Wash the apricots and cut in half. Remove the pits and chop into small pieces. Fill the measuring cup and reserve the rest for later. Set aside.

Wash the strawberries and remove the stems. Cut into small pieces and fill the measuring cup. Reserve the rest for later.

Wash the celery and chop into small pieces. Set aside.

Wash the apple and cut lengthwise in half. Remove the core and cut into small pieces. Set aside.

Now, combine apricots, strawberries, celery, and apple in a juicer and process until juiced. Transfer to a serving glass and stir in the cinnamon.

Add some ice and serve immediately.

Nutritional information per serving: Kcal: 170, Protein: 4.3g, Carbs: 49.9g, Fats: 1.4g

23.   Mint Melon Juice

Ingredients:

1 cup of watermelon, chopped

1 large banana, chopped

1 whole lime, peeled

1 cup of fresh mint, torn

1 small Granny Smith's apple, cored

¼ tsp of cinnamon, ground

Preparation:

Cut the watermelon in half. Cut one large wedge and wrap the rest in a plastic foil and refrigerate. Peel the slice and cut into small cubes. Remove the pits and fill the measuring cup. Set aside.

Peel the banana and cut into small chunks. Set aside.

Peel the lime and cut lengthwise in half. Set aside.

Wash the mint thoroughly under cold running water. Drain and torn into small pieces. Set aside.

Wash the apple and cut lengthwise in half. Remove the core and chop into bite-sized pieces. Set aside.

Now, combine watermelon, banana, lime, mint, and apple in a juicer and process until juiced. Transfer to a serving glass and stir in the cinnamon.

Add some crushed ice and serve immediately.

Nutritional information per serving: Kcal: 239, Protein: 4.2g, Carbs: 69.5g, Fats: 1.2g

24.   Brussels Sprout Artichoke Juice

Ingredients:

2 cups of Brussels sprouts, halved

1 large artichoke, chopped

1 cup of cucumber, sliced

¼ tsp of turmeric, ground

¼ tsp of ginger, ground

2 oz of water

Preparation:

Wash the Brussels sprouts and trim off the outer layers. Cut each sprout in half and fill the measuring cups. Set aside.

Trim off the outer leaves of the artichoke. Cut into small pieces and set aside.

Wash the cucumber and cut into thin slices. Fill the measuring cup and reserve the rest in the refrigerator.

Now, combine Brussels sprouts, artichoke, and cucumber in a juicer and process until well juiced. Transfer to a serving glass and stir in the ginger, turmeric, and water.

Refrigerate for 15 minutes before serving.

Enjoy!

Nutritional information per serving: Kcal: 98, Protein: 11.6g, Carbs: 34.7g, Fats: 0.8g

25.   Strawberry Pear Juice

Ingredients:

1 cup of strawberries, chopped

1 large pear, chopped

1 cup of blackberries

1 small Red Delicious apple, cored

¼ tsp of cinnamon, ground

1 oz of water

Preparation:

Wash the strawberries and remove the stems. Cut into small pieces and fill the measuring cup. Reserve the rest in the refrigerator.

Wash the pear and cut in half. Remove the core and cut into small pieces. Set aside.

Wash the blackberries using a colander. Drain and set aside.

Wash the apple and cut lengthwise in half. Remove the core and chop into bite-sized pieces. Set aside.

Now, combine strawberries, pear, blackberries, and apple in a juicer and process until well juiced. Transfer to a serving glass and stir in the cinnamon.

Refrigerate for 15 minutes before serving.

Enjoy!

Nutritional information per serving: Kcal: 246, Protein: 4.2g, Carbs: 82.1g, Fats: 1.7g

26.   Spinach Honeydew Melon Juice

Ingredients:

1 cup of spinach, chopped

1 medium-sized wedge of honeydew melon

1 cup of raspberries

1 small Golden Delicious apple, cored

¼ tsp of ginger, ground

Preparation:

Wash the spinach thoroughly under cold running water. Drain and chop into small pieces. Set aside.

Cut melon lengthwise in half. Scoop out the seeds and then wash the melon. Cut one wedge and peel it. Cut into bite-sized pieces and set aside. Reserve the rest in the refrigerator.

Place the raspberries in a colander and rinse well under cold running water. Drain and set aside.

Wash the apple and cut lengthwise in half. Remove the core and cut into bite-sized pieces. Set aside.

Now, combine spinach, melon, raspberries, and apple in a juicer and process until juiced. Transfer to a serving glass and stir in the ginger. Add some ice before serving.

Enjoy!

Nutritional information per serving: Kcal: 142, Protein: 4.5g, Carbs: 46.1g, Fats: 1.4g

27.   Orange Fennel Juice

Ingredients:

1 large orange, peeled

1 cup of fennel, chopped

1 small Granny Smith's apple, cored

1 cup of blueberries

¼ tsp of ginger, ground

Preparation:

Peel the orange and divide into wedges. Cut each wedge in half and set aside.

Trim off the outer wilted layers of the fennel. Roughly chop it and fill the measuring cup. Reserve the rest for later.

Wash the apple and cut lengthwise in half. Remove the core and cut into bite-sized pieces. Set aside.

Place the blueberries in a colander and wash thoroughly under cold running water. Drain and set aside.

Now, combine orange, fennel, apple, and blueberries in a juicer and process until juiced. Transfer to a serving glass and stir in the ginger.

Add few ice cubes and serve immediately.

Enjoy!

Nutritional information per serving: Kcal: 222, Protein: 4.5g, Carbs: 69.1g, Fats: 1.5g

28.   Raspberry Blueberry Juice

Ingredients:

2 cups of raspberries

1 cup of blueberries

1 medium-sized zucchini, sliced

1 small ginger knob, peeled

1 oz of coconut water

Preparation:

Combine raspberries and blueberries in a large colander. Rinse well under cold running water. Drain and set aside.

Wash the zucchini and cut into thin slices. Set aside.

Peel the ginger knob and cut into small pieces. Set aside.

Now, combine raspberries, blueberries, zucchini, and ginger in a juicer and process until juiced. Transfer to a serving glass and stir in the coconut water.

Add crushed ice or refrigerate for 15 minutes before serving.

Enjoy!

Nutritional information per serving: Kcal: 164, Protein: 6.5g, Carbs: 58g, Fats: 2.7g

29.   Sweet Potato Lemon Juice

Ingredients:

1 cup of sweet potato, cubed

1 whole lemon, peeled

1 cup of fresh spinach, torn

1 cup of pomegranate seeds

2 oz of water

Preparation:

Peel the sweet potato and cut into small cubes. Place in a deep pot and add 3 cups of water. Bring it to a boil and cook for 5 minutes. Remove from the heat and drain. Set aside.

Peel the lemon and cut lengthwise in half. Set aside.

Wash the spinach thoroughly under cold running water. Drain and torn into small pieces. Set aside.

Cut the top of the pomegranate fruit using a sharp paring knife. Slice down to each of the white membranes inside of the fruit. Pop the seeds into a measuring cup and set aside.

Now, combine previously cooked potato, lemon, spinach, and pomegranate seeds in a juicer. Process until well juiced.

Transfer to a serving glass and stir in the water. Add some ice and serve immediately.

Enjoy!

Nutritional information per serving: Kcal: 195, Protein: 10.2g, Carbs: 56.1g, Fats: 2.1g

30.   Broccoli Kale Juice

Ingredients:

2 cups of broccoli, chopped

2 cups of kale, chopped

1 cup of cucumber, sliced

1 whole lime, peeled and halved

1 whole lemon, peeled and halved

1 oz of water

Preparation:

Wash the broccoli and trim off the outer leaves. Cut into small pieces and fill the measuring cup. Reserve the rest in the refrigerator.

Wash the kale thoroughly under cold running water. Drain and chop into small pieces. Set aside.

Wash the cucumber and cut into thin slices. Fill the measuring cup and reserve the rest for later.

Peel the lime and lemon. Cut each fruit lengthwise in half and set aside.

Now, combine broccoli, kale, cucumber, lime, and lemon in a juicer and process until juiced. Transfer to a serving glass and stir in the water.

Sprinkle with some mint for some extra taste, but it's optional.

Refrigerate for 10 minutes before serving.

Enjoy!

Nutritional information per serving: Kcal: 116, Protein: 12.1g, Carbs: 34.8g, Fats: 2.2g

31. Mango Peach Juice

Ingredients:

1 cup of mango, chopped

1 large peach, chopped

1 whole plum, chopped

1 small Red Delicious apple, cored

1 oz of coconut water

Preparation:

Peel the mango and cut into small cubes. Fill the measuring cup and reserve the rest for later.

Wash the peach and cut lengthwise in half. Remove the pit and cut into small pieces. Set aside.

Wash the plum and cut in half. Remove the pit and chop into small pieces. Set aside.

Wash the apple cut lengthwise in half. Remove the core and chop into small pieces. Set aside.

Now, combine mango, peach, plum, and apple in a juicer and process until juiced. Transfer to a serving glass and stir in the coconut water.

Add some ice and serve immediately.

Nutritional information per serving: Kcal: 252, Protein: 3.8g, Carbs: 71.1g, Fats: 1.6g

32.   Strawberry Watermelon Juice

Ingredients:

1 cup of strawberries, chopped

1 large wedge of watermelon

1 large banana, sliced

2 whole plums, pitted

Preparation:

Wash the strawberries and remove the stems. Cut into small pieces and fill the measuring cup. Reserve the rest for in the refrigerator.

Cut the watermelon in half. Cut one large wedge and wrap the rest in a plastic foil and refrigerate. Peel the slice and cut into small cubes. Remove the pits and fill the measuring cup. Set aside.

Peel the banana and cut into thin slices. Set aside.

Wash the plums and cut into halves. Remove the pits and cut into small pieces. Set aside.

Now, combine strawberries, watermelon, banana, and plums in a juicer and process until juiced. Transfer to a serving glass and add some ice.

Serve immediately.

Nutritional information per serving: Kcal: 273, Protein: 5.1g, Carbs: 78.8g, Fats: 1.6g

33.   Cantaloupe Blackberry Juice

Ingredients:

1 cup of cantaloupe, chopped

1 cup of blackberries

2 whole kiwis, peeled

1 small green apple, cored

¼ tsp of ginger, ground

Preparation:

Cut the cantaloupe in half. Scrape out the seeds and cut one one large wedge. Peel and chop into small pieces. Wrap the rest in a plastic foil and refrigerate for later.

Place the blackberries in a colander. Rinse well under cold running water and drain. Set aside.

Peel the kiwi and cut in half. Set aside.

Wash the apple and cut lengthwise in half. Remove the core and cut into bite-sized pieces. Set aside.

Now, combine cantaloupe, blackberries, kiwi, and apple in a juicer and process until juiced. Transfer to a serving glass and stir in the ginger.

Add few ice cubes and serve immediately.

Nutritional information per serving: Kcal: 181, Protein: 4.7g, Carbs: 56.3g, Fats: 1.6g

34.   Lemon Pineapple Juice

Ingredients:

1 whole lemon, peeled

1 cup of pineapple, chunked

1 whole grapefruit, peeled and wedged

1 cup of black grapes

¼ tsp of cinnamon, ground

Preparation:

Peel the lemon and cut lengthwise in half. Set aside.

Using a sharp paring knife, cut the top of the pineapple. Gently remove all hard skin and cut into chunks. Fill the measuring cup and reserve the in the refrigerator.

Peel the grapefruit and divide into wedges. Cut each wedge in half and set aside.

Rinse the grapes thoroughly under cold running water. Remove the stems and fill the measuring cup. Set aside.

Now, combine lemon, pineapple, grapefruit, and grapes in a juicer and process until juiced. Transfer to a serving glass and stir in the cinnamon.

Add some crushed ice and serve immediately.

Nutritional information per serving: Kcal: 230, Protein: 4g, Carbs: 69.1g, Fats: 1.1g

35.   Pomegranate Blueberry Juice

Ingredients:

1 cup of pomegranate seeds

1 cup of blueberries

1 whole lime, peeled

1 small Granny Smith's apple, cored

¼ tsp of ginger, ground

2 oz of water

Preparation:

Cut the top of the pomegranate fruit using a sharp paring knife. Slice down to each of the white membranes inside of the fruit. Pop the seeds into a measuring cup and set aside.

Place the blueberries in a colander. Rinse well under cold running water and drain. Set aside.

Peel the lime and cut lengthwise in half. Set aside.

Wash the apple and cut lengthwise in half. Remove the core and cut into bite-sized pieces and set aside.

Now, combine pomegranate seeds, blueberries, lime, and apple in a juicer and process until juiced. Transfer to a serving glass and stir in the ginger and water.

Refrigerate for 10 minutes before serving.

Enjoy!

Nutritional information per serving: Kcal: 206, Protein: 3.3g, Carbs: 61.1g, Fats: 1.8g

36. Peach Beet Juice

Ingredients:

1 large peach, pitted and chopped

1 cup of beets, trimmed and sliced

1 cup of apricots, sliced

1 whole lemon, peeled and halved

1 small ginger slice, peeled

1 oz of water

Preparation:

Wash the peach and cut lengthwise in half. Remove the pit and chop into bite-sized pieces. Set aside.

Wash the beets and trim off the green ends. Slightly peel and cut into thin slices. Fill the measuring cup and reserve the rest for later.

Wash the apricots and cut lengthwise in half. Remove the pits and cut into thin slices. Fill the measuring cup and reserve the rest in the refrigerator.

Peel the ginger slice and chop into small pieces. Set aside.

Now, combine peach, beets, apricots, lemon, and ginger in a juicer and process until juiced. Transfer to a serving glass and stir in the water.

Refrigerate for 15 minutes before serving.

Nutritional information per serving: Kcal: 180, Protein: 6.7g, Carbs: 53.8g, Fats: 1.5g

37. Apple Cherry Juice

Ingredients:

1 small Golden Delicious apple, cored

1 cup of cherries

1 cup of celery, chopped

1 whole plum, pitted and chopped

¼ tsp of cinnamon, ground

2 tbsp of coconut water

Preparation:

Wash the apple and cut lengthwise in half. Remove the core and cut into bite-sized pieces. Set aside.

Wash the cherries using a colander. Drain and cut each in half. Remove the pits and set aside.

Now, combine apple, cherries, celery, and plum in a juicer and process until juiced. Transfer to a serving glass and stir in the cinnamon and coconut water.

Add some crushed ice and serve immediately.

Nutritional information per serving: Kcal: 182, Protein: 3.1g, Carbs: 52.7g, Fats: 0.8g

38. Fennel Bell Pepper Juice

Ingredients:

1 cup of fennel, sliced

1 large yellow bell pepper, chopped

1 cup of Romaine lettuce, chopped

1 cup of cucumber, sliced

1 small zucchini, cubed

Preparation:

Trim off the fennel bulb and remove the green parts. Wash it and cut into small pieces. Fill the measuring cup and reserve the rest for later. Set aside.

Wash the bell pepper and cut lengthwise in half. Remove the stem and seeds. Cut into small pieces and set aside.

Wash the Romaine lettuce thoroughly under cold running water. Drain and chop into small pieces. Set aside.

Wash the cucumber and cut into thin slices. Fill the measuring cup and reserve the rest for later.

Wash the zucchini and cut into small cubes. Set aside.

Now, combine fennel, bell pepper, lettuce, cucumber, and zucchini in a juicer and process until juiced. Transfer to a serving glass and refrigerate for 10 minutes before serving.

Nutritional information per serving: Kcal: 85, Protein: 5.3g, Carbs: 25.2g, Fats: 1.1g

39.   Tomato Asparagus Juice

Ingredients:

1 medium-sized tomato, chopped

1 cup of asparagus, trimmed and chopped

1 cup of collard greens, torn

1 cup of spinach, torn

¼ tsp salt

1 rosemary sprig

Preparation:

Wash the tomato and place it in a small bowl. Cut into small pieces and reserve the tomato juice while cutting. Set aside.

Wash the asparagus and trim off the woody ends. Cut into small pieces and fill the measuring cup. Set aside.

Combine collard greens and spinach in a large colander. Wash under cold running water and drain. Torn into small pieces and set aside.

Now, combine tomato, asparagus, collard greens, and spinach in a juicer and process until juiced. Transfer to a serving glass and stir in the reserve tomato juice and salt. Sprinkle with rosemary.

You can add some basil for some extra taste, but it's optional.

Serve immediately.

Nutritional information per serving: Kcal: 66, Protein: 11.2g, Carbs: 19.6g, Fats: 1.5g

40.   Orange Broccoli Juice

Ingredients:

1 large orange, peeled

1 cup of broccoli, chopped

1 cup of cucumber, sliced

1 whole lime, peeled and halved

2 oz of coconut water

¼ tsp of ginger, ground

Preparation:

Peel the orange and divide into wedges. Cut each wedge in half and set aside.

Wash the broccoli and trim off the outer leaves. Cut into small pieces and fill the measuring cup. Reserve the rest in the refrigerator.

Wash the cucumber and cut into thin slices. Fill the measuring cup and reserve the rest for later.

Peel the lime and cut lengthwise in half. Set aside.

Now, combine orange, broccoli, cucumber, and lime in a juicer and process until juiced. Transfer to a serving glass and stir in the coconut water and ginger. Add some ice and serve immediately.

Nutritional information per serving: Kcal: 106, Protein: 4.8g, Carbs: 33.3g, Fats: 0.6g

41.   Guava Strawberry Juice

Ingredients:

1 whole guava, chunked

1 cup of strawberries, chopped

1 small Granny Smith's apple, cored and chopped

1 whole lemon, peeled and halved

¼ tsp of ginger, ground

2 oz of water

Preparation:

Peel the guava and cut in half. Scoop out the seeds and wash it. Cut into small chunks and set aside.

Wash the strawberries and remove the stems. Cut into small pieces and fill the measuring cup. Reserve the rest in the refrigerator. Set aside.

Wash the apple and cut lengthwise in half. Remove the core and cut into bite-sized pieces. Set aside.

Peel the lemon and cut lengthwise in half. Set aside.

Now, combine guava, strawberries, apple, and lemon in a juicer and process until juiced. Transfer to a serving glass and stir in the ginger and water.

Refrigerate for 15 minutes before serving.

Enjoy!

Nutritional information per serving: Kcal: 136, Protein: 3.6g, Carbs: 43.9g, Fats: 1.3g

42.   Banana Mint Juice

Ingredients:

2 large bananas, peeled and chopped

1 cup of fresh mint, torn

1 whole kiwi, peeled

1 whole lemon, peeled

1 large Red Delicious apple, cored and chopped

¼ tsp of cinnamon, ground

Preparation:

Peel the bananas and cut into small pieces. Set aside.

Wash the mint thoroughly under cold running water. Drain and torn into small pieces. Set aside.

Wash the apple and cut lengthwise in half. Remove the core and cut into bite-sized pieces. Set aside.

Now, combine bananas, mint, kiwi, lemon, and apple in a juicer and process until well juiced. Transfer to a serving glass and stir in the cinnamon.

Add some ice and serve immediately.

Enjoy!

Nutritional information per serving: Kcal: 398, Protein: 6.1g, Carbs: 117g, Fats: 2.1g

43.   Carrot Celery Juice

Ingredients:

2 large carrots, chunked

1 cup of celery, chopped

1 whole grapefruit, peeled

1 small Golden Delicious apple, cored and chopped

¼ tsp of cinnamon, ground

Preparation:

Wash and peel the carrots. Cut into small chunks and set aside.

Wash the celery and cut into small pieces. Fill the measuring cup and reserve the rest in the refrigerator.

Peel the grapefruit and divide into wedges. Cut each wedge in half and set aside.

Wash the apple and cut lengthwise in half. Remove the core and cut into bite-sized pieces. Set aside.

Now, combine carrots, celery, grapefruit, and apple in a juicer and process until well juiced. Transfer to a serving glass and stir in the cinnamon.

Add some crushed ice and serve immediately.

Enjoy!

Nutritional information per serving: Kcal: 203, Protein: 4.3g, Carbs: 60.6g, Fats: 1.1g

44.　Leek Pear Juice

Ingredients:

1 whole leek, chopped

1 medium-sized pear, chopped

1 whole lime, peeled

1 cup of cantaloupe, peeled and chopped

1 oz of coconut water

¼ tsp of ginger, ground

Preparation:

Wash the leek thoroughly under cold running water. Drain and chop into small pieces. Set aside.

Wash the pear lengthwise in half. Remove the core and cut into bite-sized pieces. Set aside.

Peel the lime and cut lengthwise in half. Set aside.

Cut the cantaloupe in half. Scoop out the seeds and flesh. Cut and peel one large wedge. Chop into chunks and fill the measuring cup. Reserve the rest of the cantaloupe in a refrigerator.

Now, combine leek, pear, lime, and cantaloupe in a juicer and process until juiced. Transfer to a serving glass and stir in the coconut water and ginger.

Add some ice, or refrigerate for 10 minutes before serving.

Nutritional information per serving: Kcal: 184, Protein: 3.5g, Carbs: 56.2g, Fats: 0.8g

45.   Artichoke Basil Juice

Ingredients:

1 medium-sized artichoke, chopped

1 cup of fresh basil, torn

1 cup of red leaf lettuce, chopped

1 cup of purple cabbage, chopped

1 cup of cucumber, sliced

1 large carrot, sliced

Preparation:

Trim off the outer layers of the artichoke using a sharp paring knife. Cut into bite-sized pieces and set aside.

Rinse the basil with cold water and torn into small pieces. Set aside.

Combine lettuce and cabbage in a large colander and rinse well under cold running water. Drain and chop into small pieces. Set aside.

Wash the cucumber and cut into thin slices. Fill the measuring cup and reserve the rest in the refrigerator.

Wash and peel the carrot. Cut into thin slices and set aside.

Now, combine artichoke, basil, lettuce, cabbage, cucumber, and carrot in a juicer and process until juiced. Transfer to a serving glass and serve immediately.

Nutritional information per serving: Kcal: 88, Protein: 7.6g, Carbs: 30.1g, Fats: 0.7g

46.   Avocado Plum Juice

Ingredients:

1 cup of avocado, cubed

2 whole plums, chopped

1 whole lime, pitted and chopped

1 small pear, chopped

2 oz of coconut water

¼ tsp of ginger, ground

Preparation:

Peel the avocado and cut lengthwise in half. Remove the pit and cut into small cubes. Fill the measuring cup and reserve the rest for later.

Wash the plums and cut in half. Remove the pits and cut into small pieces. Set aside.

Peel the lime and cut lengthwise in half. Set aside.

Wash the pear and cut in half. Remove the core and into bite-sized pieces. Set side.

Now, combine avocado, plums, lime, and pear in a juicer and process until juiced. Transfer to a serving glass and stir in the coconut water and ginger.

Add some ice and serve immediately.

Nutritional information per serving: Kcal: 328, Protein: 4.6g, Carbs: 54.1g, Fats: 22.6g

47. Brussels Sprout Carrot Juice

Ingredients:

2 cups of Brussels sprouts, halved

2 large radishes, chopped

1 small zucchini, chopped

1 cup of cucumber, sliced

2 large carrots, sliced

¼ tsp of turmeric, ground

Preparation:

Wash the Brussels sprouts and trim off the outer layers. Cut into halves and fill the measuring cups. Reserve the rest in the refrigerator.

Wash the radishes and trim off the green parts. Slightly peel and cut into small pieces. Set aside.

Wash the zucchini and cut into thin slices. Set aside.

Wash the cucumber and cut into thin slices. Fill the measuring cup and reserve the rest for later.

Wash and peel the carrots. Cut into thin slices and set aside.

Now, combine Brussels sprouts, radishes, zucchini, cucumber, and carrots in a juicer and process until juiced. Transfer to a serving glass and stir in the turmeric. Refrigerate for 15 minutes before serving.

Nutritional information per serving: Kcal: 118, Protein: 9.2g, Carbs: 35.7g, Fats: 1.3g

ADDITIONAL TITLES FROM THIS AUTHOR

70 Effective Meal Recipes to Prevent and Solve Being Overweight: Burn Fat Fast by Using Proper Dieting and Smart Nutrition

By

Joe Correa CSN

48 Acne Solving Meal Recipes: The Fast and Natural Path to Fixing Your Acne Problems in Less Than 10 Days!

By

Joe Correa CSN

41 Alzheimer's Preventing Meal Recipes: Reduce or Eliminate Your Alzheimer's Condition in 30 Days or Less!

By

Joe Correa CSN

70 Effective Breast Cancer Meal Recipes: Prevent and Fight Breast Cancer with Smart Nutrition and Powerful Foods

By

Joe Correa CSN

www.ingramcontent.com/pod-product-compliance
Lightning Source LLC
Chambersburg PA
CBHW030258030426
42336CB00009B/437